The World That Revolves Around Hydrocephalus

Hydrocephalus and Kacee

I0407542

Cathy Barnes & Kacee Barnes

The World That Revolves Around Hydrocephalus
Cathy Barnes and Kacee Barnes

© 2017 Cathy Barnes & Kacee Barnes

ISBN-13: 978-1545125090

ISBN- 10: 1545125090

Published by Broken Bars Publishing

www.brokenbarspublishing.com

Printed in the United States of America

Cure

I wish there were a cure for me

To be what I want to be

How could this be

God, don't you love me?

I know that we are not supposed

To question God

But why don't you have a cure

For me?

All I ask is just to be me

Not today, not tomorrow

But someday

See

The World That Revolves Around Hydrocephalus
Cathy Barnes and Kacee Barnes

My name is Kacee, I am Twenty-eight years of age, and I live with hydrocephalus. I live with what is called Dandy-Walker syndrome, which is associated with hydrocephalus (hydrocephalus-associated). The word comes from the Greek hydro, meaning water and cephalous meaning head; it is from this meaning that the phrase water-head came into being. Hydrocephalus is an abnormal accumulation of cerebrospinal fluid, or CSF. There are other reasons as to why children are born with hydrocephalus.

I was diagnosed with Dandy-Walker syndrome because my fourth ventricle was not fully developed at birth. This is my reason for the association with hydrocephalus, or water-head. You may have heard the phrase before; I know I have. There were children, at least three, that had called me water-head several times. I had no idea how they knew, but I knew I did not like it.

Everyone has his or her own struggles; I certainly have mine. As I continue my struggles throughout my life, I have come to realize that other people have inspired and strengthened me to continue on and complain less. It is clear to me that my problem seems to be only superficial compared to those of other people who have already decided to continue on anyway. This is very good for all who have.

I hope that you will get a better understanding of, at least a little more knowledge of, this syndrome and how it affects people. There are certain problems associated with this disease that gave me reasons for trying to share this part of my life with other people.

I had not read or heard of this condition outside of the neurologist's office. I needed information about this hydrocephalus-associated disease. There was something going on with me, and I needed information. I did not know how I was even feeling, what I was feeling, and more importantly, if these feelings were normal. I wanted to know about the fears I was having. Do these fears affect every person with hydrocephalus the same way? I was damaged, and I wanted to be fixed, or to know if I could be fixed, or even to know why I could not be fixed.

I wanted to rise above this disability and continue on to what I will be happy doing in my life. This is not a big autobiography, because I am not a big person. By that, I mean I have been back and forth to the hospital all my life probably more than a lot of you even go to a job. I have felt for a long time now that my life has been on hold for years. Well, get ready, world! Here I come!

This is my story, I was diagnosed with Dandy-Walker Syndrome at my six-month-old medical checkup. It was the first time that my dad had taken me to the doctor for a checkup by himself. The pediatric nurse discovered that my head was much larger than it should have been. Everything started right away. My dad called my mom, the doctor started doing tests on me, and my mom says that's when all hell broke loose. They took x-rays, did CT scans, did blood work, and also tested my motor skills. My mom arrived very soon after the tests were started.

The neurologist arrived shortly after my mom did. He informed my parents just what was going on. He told my parents that I had hydrocephalus. He said that he was still running tests to see exactly why I had hydrocephalus is the surgical placement of a shunt. My parents said that we were at the hospital pretty much the whole day. We were finally told to come back the next day, early. My parents figured that the results of the tests should be ready by morning.

When we returned the next day, the results of all the tests were back; the nurse told us that the doctor would be in soon. The neurologist came in and told us about the tests that were run. He said that the results of all the tests were within the normal ranges except for the CT scan. The CT scan told him that the fourth ventricle was not fully developed, and that cerebrospinal fluid in my brain could not be absorbed. He told us that this condition is called Dandy-Walker Syndrome. He gave my parents a short history about how this syndrome was named after it was discovered. Two doctors discovered the association to hydrocephalus by the nonfunctioning of the fourth ventricle. These doctors were Dr. Walter E. Dandy (U.S. neurosurgeon); it is from the names of these doctors that the condition Dandy Walker Syndrome was named.

The neurosurgeon was called, and we all met. He confirmed the fact that I had Dandy-Walker Syndrome. He also explained the shunt and how it works. The shunt is a long plastic tube that allows fluid to drain from the brain to another part of the body, the abdomen. The shunt was called the VP shunt; the ventricular peritoneal shunt would be what was used for me. The shunt would start from the upper back side of the brain, to the large vein in the neck, and down to the abdomen. He wanted us to know that the placement of the shunt does not cure hydrocephalus; hydrocephalus is a lifelong illness.

My parents told me that there was so much information that they had to digest, in such a short amount of time, that it was very scary. They were able to understand that this was a chronic condition, and that future for me would include doctors and hospitals from then on. Both of my parents told me that it was not about what I needed for the future. It was about my having a future, whether it was healthy or compromised. Whatever was needed, my parents decided that nothing was too much or me to have in life. The neurosurgeon gave us surgery date, and we were right there on time. It took a long time to get checked in for surgery.

I was put into the room that I would be in for the rest of my stay in the hospital. My parents have told me many times the story about the time I had surgery, but I always like to hear it again. I was admitted to my room, with monitors and IV tubes, three days before surgery. My parents told me all about the pressures they were feeling on the day of my surgery. It was the fourth day when I went to surgery. I was told that my parents paid very close attention to what was happening that fourth day. The nurses came in to give medication to me, and, of course, I did not want to take it. Nevertheless, they did get it down me anyway. They told me that that I started getting drowsy right away. The doctor came in to see my parents and also to see how I was reacting to the meds. After he finished reassuring them that there was nothing to worry about, he left to get ready for surgery. Soon after that, surgery personnel came to get me. My parents remember seeing me disappear down the hall and how frightened they were at that moment. They told me that after that, the clock seemed to have stopped, and time seemed to stand still.

Everything from then on went very slowly for the rest of the day. I was in surgery for at least three to four hours, and they said that those three to four hours felt like an eternity. After the surgery was completed, my doctor came to let them know that I would be back in my room; they came to let them know that I would be back in my room; they came to meet me as I was being rolled down the hall in my crib. The first thing they saw was the bandage on my head. The doctor came back to explain things. He told them that everything went according to plan, that there were no problems then, and also that he did not expect any problems afterward. He was quite optimistic about my recovery.

My mom wanted to hold me as soon as I was put back in my crib. The doctor explained to us that I had to lie at a forty-five-degree angle and that I was not to be picked up, because my brain had to settle slowly. It would be two weeks before they were able to hold me.

My mom said that she was so glad that she got a chance to hold me all day before surgery; she said that she felt so much better with me in her arms. Now this bombshell news made it hard to do. That was a shock to her system, and so unexpected.

My parents told me how they communicated with me. They told me that I would grab their fingers, one at a time. And I would shake their finger like I was shaking their hand. My mom told me that not being able to hold me was one of the hardest things she had to do. She told me that her arms were aching to hold me, and that two weeks took a long time to get there. When the time came, she wanted to hold me so bad that she held me all night long and into the next day. After surgery was over, my mom says that I really worked hard to recover; everything was a struggle for me. She said that even though the road for me was tough, I kept the fight up, and my recovery was clearly visible just days after surgery.

It was just a matter of time before I would regain my health, and come back to just about 100 percent of where I was in the beginning. She told me that I made the whole fight process appear to look like a very smooth operation. I had a tough fight, they told me, but they knew I would make it through. Th doctor had quite a lot of information that we needed to now information pertaining to health-care changes for my life. He told us that there are certain warning signs to be on the lookout for. When the shunt malfunctions, signs to be on the lookout for. When the shunt malfunctions, signs tell us that the shunt is not working properly. Signs to look for are a headache that gets worse as time passes, vomiting, or feeling sick to the stomach, changes in personality, not being alert, loss of mental and physical abilities, and vision problems.

Other signs to watch for are signs of a shunt infection: a fever that is 100.4 degrees or higher, redness or swelling of the skin along the path of the VP shunt, or pain around the shunt or around the shunt tubing. We were to contact the doctor right away even if we suspected that something might or might not be wrong. My parents said that these instructions were a little scary at first; however, they felt that together they were capable and strong enough to handle this delicate situation for their daughter's sake. My dad told me that because the cerebrospinal fluid could not be absorbed, there was nowhere for it to go, so it kept building up inside my head.

When the fluid would build up in my head, it would push my brain up, and that would cause pain in my head when I would smile. To keep the pain away, I would look down, because it felt better for my head. When I did smile, my dad said he knew that the fluid was being absorbed the way it was supposed to. He still smiles every time I laugh or smile.

I stayed in the hospital for forty-five days; I am so sure that I was happy to go home. I was told that my medical reports said that at the time of my six-month-old checkup, I was normal and doing what a normal 7-month-old baby was supposed to be doing. I was developing at a normal pace. Now, after surgery, my parents were being told to watch for signs of abnormal development and/or behavior.

When I came home after surgery, I was making what the doctors called, "Good progress." My progress was right on time; in fact, it was better than on time. My doctor was very satisfied. I was told that I started walking at eleven months old. My vocabulary was at a normal daily rate, and I was using my right hand at all times, as my parents made sure I did. Within the next year, there were few to no problems with my health. Except for an occasional headache, there were no other worries. I had appointments at least two times a month with the neurologists who kept close tabs on me. My weight was low, but still healthy. My head was within a normal circumference, and my height was short. However, most people with hydrocephalus are short in stature.

I always played in my mom's shoes, and I had tea parties with my green tea set. I would tell my mom to let me get my own high heel shoes since I loved playing in her shoes so much.

When I was two years old, I remember getting headaches that I would tell my mom about. I remember one day when my headache was so bad it made me go to the doctor. Later I ended up going to the hospital. Just because I can remember these instances, I don't mean that I can recall everything that happened to me at two years old.

My mom had finally decided to take me shopping to find shoes like hers. I had a headache that day, but I thought it might go away. I tried to ignore it, because I wanted those shoes. I saw shoes, but there were no red shoes like the ones I wanted. I asked the salesman if they had any red shoes in my size. The salesman told us that he did not have any, but there might be red shoes at the toy store. My mom took me to the toy store. There they were. The red high heels that I had wanted for so long. I just knew I would have twinkle toes when I put these shoes on.

My head continued to hurt, but I still wanted to try the shoes on. After I tried them on, I took them off right away. I told my mom that my head was hurting and my mom picked me up with the shoes and carried me to the car. I laid down until we got home. I did not want to play or anything. I just wanted to go to bed. My mom laid down with me so that she could see if my condition got worse during the night. My dad was working the late shift and was not home. I was lying there feeling sick when I heard my mom snore. I wanted to go to the bathroom, but I was afraid to go alone. I called out my mom's name, but she was still snoring and did not wake up. So, I got my flashlight and went to the bathroom by myself. When I came back, I shined the light right into my mom's face, but she never woke up. The next morning when I woke up, I wanted to play dress up and have a tea party with my favorite tea set.

I thought I had been up for a while, but my mom told me I had only been up about 10 minutes. My head started to hurt again really bad. I suddenly did not want to play twinkle toes anymore. I did not even want to have a tea party. I was on my way to lie down, and the next thing I remember, I was at the hospital getting tests done. I was in this large X-ray looking machine that was recording what was happening as I was getting a needle in my back. My mom told me that I had a seizure, or what she believed to be a seizure. She also told me that the doctor reported this was not a shunt-related problem; he had already ruled out shunt malfunction. Instead I was diagnosed with migraine headaches and hospitalized for nine days.

I was very happy to go home. When I walked in, there were lots of balloons waiting for me. The children from my nursery school had made get well cards for me. I rested for a week before going back to school. I was happy to get back return, and my classmates were happy to see me come back also.

I was back to having fun soon after I returned home, playing dress-up, wearing those twinkle-toe red high heels and having my tea parties again. There were new instructions and medications now. The instructions had the same things to look out for, only the wording was a little different.

I turned three years old shortly after I returned home from the hospital. I got lots of balloons and presents. I really liked that part. What I remember most about that summer was the peach tree we had out back. I would get out in the early mornings and pick green peaches. I liked the green peaches, and though my dad did not want me eating them, my mom would let me because she liked the peaches too. Sometimes we even picked them together.

My mom washed and dried the fruit as we sat in the breakfast room eating green peaches with vinegar, seasoned salt, and pepper. My dad got up at about 6:30 a.m. came into the kitchen and asked what was I eating. My mom told him it was green peaches with vinegar, seasoned salt, and pepper. He said, "This early? Why don't you just give her a bucket of gasoline for breakfast?"

"Gasoline might be good with green peaches. Maybe we will try that next time Kacee," my mom said as she and my dad laughed.

Mom got up to answer the phone. As she left the room, she said, "Don't drink all of my vinegar. And by no means should you eat all of her peaches."

I laughed, at the both of them. Thinking back, that was a good summer.

It took some time for me to finally be able to do things on my own. It seemed like forever. I think I was becoming a different person. I was still dressing up in my red high heel twinkle-toe shoes, and I still having tea

12

parties, but I knew that things had changed. I got a new bedroom with a bed like everyone else had. My room was not a baby room anymore, even though I still played with my toys. I started to realize, I was not a baby anymore.

For my fourth birthday, I got a game called Tempest. It was a very big game. I had to stand on a footstool when I wanted to play it. I played that game until I learned to reach high levels. After I would get past the highest level of the game, the Tempest game would prompt me to write my name next to the highest level.

I remember also that around this time, I would put a couple of pecans outside on the back porch, and a squirrel would come and get them. I did this all the time. One day, I was watching something on the breakfast room TV and forgot to put pecans out. I heard something fall on the back porch, but I paid no attention to the noise. After a few minutes, I heard something fall again. When I went out to investigate the strange noises at the back door, I saw the squirrel standing there on its hind legs, begging with its hands. This was the same squirrel that came every day. Now it knocked things down to get my attention. I threw a few pecans out to it just as I always had. The squirrel grabbed one and left.

I was five years old when I first encountered that squirrel. It had been over twenty years now, and that squirrel still comes up on the back porch, knocks something down, waits, and begs with its hands while standing on its hind legs. I throw pecans out, it grabs them, and runs off.

I always thought it was only one squirrel, but my mom said it was a bunch of squirrels. My dad would say that mom didn't know what she is talking about that she thought she knew everything. He said to just ignore her, and maybe she'll go away. My mom would say, "He's right. She does know everything." They would both laugh and I would say, "There sure are a lot of squirrels that know how to come to the back porch, knock and beg."

Right about that time, I thought that they both thought they knew everything. One squirrel started to come into the back door, but never went past the washer/dryer. It's true.

My mom would say that these are hood squirrels. They don't even know how to store food up for the winter, like squirrels we read about in books. She'd say that they needed help. My dad would say that she was right. That was one of the few issues that they agreed on. My dad would say that the squirrels can't see where they bury the nuts anyway.

I wrote a letter to Romper Room, a show taped in Hollywood that came on channel 13. I received an invitation to appear on the show shortly after I sent the letter. I remember I had to go there for two days of filming since the show aired five days a week. On the first day, they recorded two episodes. On the second day, they filmed for three episodes. I changed my clothes for each different episode.

I met several five year olds that were on the show with me. We all had fun with the Romper Room teacher. We had class every day where we learned shapes, colors and numbers. We did crafts and played games. On the fifth day, we graduated. I said goodbye to the children, and I have never seen any of them again.

I remember at about this same time, as soon as I would come home from school, the first thing I would do was to look for some birds that had just started to come around lately. Someone had dressed two birds up in clothes. One had on a tuxedo, a vest, and a red bow tie. The other bird had on what looked like a coat to me. My mom said it was a coat dress. However, my dad said they both had on tuxedos. Everyone in the neighborhood was wondering where the pigeons had come from, and who would have dressed them up this way. I watched the birds every day until they stopped coming back. I was a little sad when they did not return.

My mom said that the birds had come around for about three months, but my dad said it was only about two and a half months. My mom said that she had written the date down. My dad did not know what to say after that. As of today, my father and I have never seen any documentation pertaining to the length of time these two birds stayed. We ended up calling the birds the "Hollywood Birds."

Of course, no one ever believed any of our stories about the two birds. But what can I say? It's true.

As the years went by, there were family events that took place that were recorded as family history. My uncle was getting married, and the wedding was going to be a big one. I was the flower girl in this very large wedding, and after two rehearsals, I was sure that I could do my part right when it was time for the wedding. When the day finally arrived, and it was my turn to go down the aisle, I tried to walk just right, so that I would not walk too fast or too slow, dropping flowers as I walked. I moved carefully so that I would drop the flowers in just the right spots. This was the first time I had ever been in a wedding, and I was very serious about my part. While the ceremony was going on, I could only think, I want this kind of wedding one day when I get married. By the time everything was over, I was very tired, but I was glad I had done my part right.

I should have thought, if I get married, instead of when. Because it does not look as if I will ever get married.

But just in case my Mister Right is out there, somewhere, that is the kind of wedding we will have.

I was having headaches from time to time, but I was never really afraid of them. I thought they were normal, so I tried to ignore them. They got so bad that I was no longer able to ignore them. It was then that I began to be afraid that something might happen. Something that I wouldn't be able to control.

Every year on Martin Luther King's Birthday, we would plant a tree or a flower and barbeque. When I was eight years old, I was sitting out back watching my dad barbeque, as I tried to get over a headache. As I sat there, a bird came down and took a chicken leg right off the grill. My mom was standing there, and said, "Did you see that bird take that piece of chicken, Kacee?" I said yes. My dad said that it was a hawk. "Did you see how all the birds got out the way, when that hawk first came down? Can you see how much bigger it is than the other birds?" We saw that all the other birds stayed away as long as the hawk was around. I was so busy watching the hawk scare the other birds, that I forgot I was sick.

I had just turned ten years old, when Nana, my great grandmother died. After her funeral, I didn't know if I would ever be able to go on. I loved Nana so much, and have never stopped missing her. Nana's funeral was so painful for me, that I noticed the stress from the event triggered more reoccurring episodes of the same headaches I was dealing with all the time.

The headaches would last two, three, and sometimes four days. It felt as though someone had dropped a brick on my head. The headaches would cause my body to become paralyzed on my right side. That made me even more afraid of the headaches. It was why I dealt with the bad headaches right away.

The medication I took was very hard on me. Sometimes it worked, and sometimes it didn't. Sometimes I got sick, and sometimes I didn't. Sometimes it made me sleepy, and sometimes it wouldn't. Well, so much for medication!

I did science projects and reports in school. I had some difficulties, but I got through it okay. I kept looking out for learning disabilities in myself. I thought that by the time I had reached age eleven, I would be able to see my own disabilities. I could not. I did, however, start having abnormalities in my vision. I started seeing circles all the time, which was very annoying to me. My mom took me to the doctor to see what was wrong. When he did not see anything wrong, I became even more annoyed.

It was time for the family reunion. Gram had received the information and faxed it to us. The family reunion was going to be in New Orleans this time. I was so excited, because I had wanted to go to Mardi Gras for a long time.

I still had my braces on, and I did not like that one bit. It seemed as though I had those braces on from birth. So, when it was time to go the reunion, I decided to get different bands or something other than what I had.

I was so excited that I could not sleep too well before the reunion. Preparing for a trip is just as exciting as the trip itself, to me. Anyway, I could not wait for the day. Our family reunions took place every other year, in a different city. Sometimes when I would see where it was going to be, I would say that I did not want to go there. But guess what? I was always glad that I went after all.

Since my mom and dad didn't care much to travel, Gram and Grandad always took me to the reunion. I started getting my stuff ready to go to New Orleans early. I am so blessed to have my grandparents. I love them dearly.

After we arrived in New Orleans, we went straight to the rental car place where the car was already waiting for us. When we got to the hotel we put our things up. Since we were early, we got into the Town Car and drove around to see things. I started looking out the window as Gram drove through the streets. As we drove, I felt something on my leg, but I just kept looking out of the window. When I finally looked down, I saw a lizard on my leg.

"There's a lizard on my leg," I said.

"What!" Gram said, as she pulled over to the curb.

"There is a lizard on my leg," I said again.

By the time, Gram was parked. I was shaking as we all jumped out of the car.

Grandad checked the back seat and got the lizard out. When we saw it, we thought to never forget to check a rental car before we got into it. Now that I look back on that incident, it seems a little funny, however, I can tell you that there was nothing funny that day.

When we arrived back at our hotel room, we only had enough time to freshen up and meet the family for dinner. Here we were at this family function, where music, stories, and memories were happening. The first event is when family members connect with other family members whom they have never met or whom they have not seen in many years. It is our opening ceremony. My favorite activity of our reunion.

We returned home safely, and let me tell you, there is no place like home.

My mom made a doctor's appointment for me the next day. I told the doctor about the spell I had while I was in New Orleans. He checked me for any signs or problems I may have had. He saw nothing wrong. I had no shunt malfunction.

I went to the doctor two more times with the same problem, and they still found nothing wrong. No shunt malfunction. I kept thinking, there has to be something wrong. I could feel that something wasn't right. I knew that after twelve years, I was in trouble again. Symptoms were back that told me surgery had to be done again.

My brother was having a wedding soon. So I got caught up into the mix of that, and tried not to let my problem get in the way. I was a bridesmaid in the wedding, and by the time the wedding came around, I had started to gain weight and was always tired after walking short distances.

I have always weighed eighty-nine pounds, even with my clothes and shoes on. My mom even noticed symptoms I was having. That is when we both knew something was wrong. My mom asked me if I wanted to go to the doctor. I said I would wait until the wedding was over.

The wedding day was very beautiful. Everyone looked great, and the reception was lovely. I was surprised to have remained headache free throughout the whole day, even though it was an extremely long day for me. I was just sorry that I was not able to give the wedding my full attention. During the event, all I could think of was that I wanted to tell my mom to take me to the doctor right away. My mom took me to the doctor the very next day.

The doctor examined me and asked me if I was pregnant. I told him, "Not until I am married." He then looked for irregular pupils, disturbed thoughts or behavior, weakness in my limbs, and raised pressure within the skull. Everything appeared to be okay, according to the doctor. He then tapped on my back and on my stomach. He did some other things also, and told us that there was fluid that had accumulated. He said he didn't know why I was retaining fluid, but he was admitting me to the hospital right away.

I was given an ID bracelet and a hospital gown to put on. A nurse put an IV line in my arm drew blood, took my blood pressure and my temperature. The hospital performed blood tests, CT, and MRI scans, and x ray exams.

By the time, I got to a room, I was so worried. It was clear to me that my body was telling me that I really did need to have surgery. I got really scared, because every time I have a shunt malfunction, there is a need for surgery. Every time there is surgery, there is a possibility of brain damage. That is a very stressful thought that I had as I thought of the surgery.

I had no idea of just what was what. All I knew was that I had been admitted and that my doctor was not even there. He wouldn't be there for at least another four days. The admitting doctor came into my room to extract fluid from my stomach, so that medical tests could be run on it. He injected a large needle into my stomach and withdrew two five-hundred-milliliter containers of cerebrospinal fluid. I could not believe that I actually felt relieved after that. The admitting doctor took care of me daily until my surgeon returned from vacation. I had been in the hospital for four days before I saw my doctor.

When my doctor returned, he verified the fact that I did need surgery. He told us that my body was no longer absorbing the fluid as it had done in the past. He did not know why this had happened, but it needed to be fixed right away. He told us that he had to reroute the VP shunt tubing from the right side of my chest to a VA shunt in my left lung space.

After he told me that I had to have surgery, my hands started to sweat. I felt like my life had just ended. Even though I knew the surgery was the only way I was going to get better, I still did not want to deal with the scary part of the surgery itself. Surgery is one of the scariest things that a person can go through.

The night before surgery, I was not to have anything to eat after midnight. First thing the morning of the surgery, I was given a small white pill to take to help to relax me, which is exactly what it did. A little while later, someone came to my room to pick me up for surgery. My mom and dad kissed me goodbye. I had taken my baby troll with me as they wheeled me down the hallway to the operating room.

Once I was inside, my doctor shaved my head. I was then given oxygen and an anesthetic, and told to count back from one hundred. I started the count and the next thing I remember, the nurse was waking me up from the anesthesia, and telling me that they were taking me back to my room. My throat was very sore, I was so sleepy that I could hardly keep my eyes open.

The next time I opened my eyes, the first thing I saw were my parents' faces. There were still blood tests that my doctor had ordered. I had to give more blood for the tests. When the phlebotomist came into my room to draw more blood, I ran into the bathroom and called my mom. I did all that, and I still had to get my blood drawn.

Weeks after surgery, the doctor had come to the conclusion that it was time for me to finally get out of the hospital. It felt so good to have the IV line out of my arm. When I got discharged, a nurse wheeled me out to the car in a chair. They gave us instructions to return in three days in order to have the staples removed from my head. I asked the doctor what I should look out for, and how long the surgery would last. He told me that no one really knows the long term effects on hydrocephalus patients.

It had been forty days since I was admitted to the hospital. I could not wait to be home in the confines of my own living quarters. There really is no place like home. Now I had to get on with the business of recuperation. I had little things that I needed to do in order to get better. I had a little tool I had to inhale two times a day. Also, there were two exercises I had to do on a daily basis. I was even home schooled during my recuperation period.

I tried to become more involved in church and participated in church activities. I was a member of the usher board, and I enjoyed spiritual dancing. But my body couldn't handle the activities so I was unable to continue.

I had participated in a Beautillion Ball for another church. I was invited to attend with a young man from that church. The Beautillion was a very beautiful ceremony in which the young man dedicated his life to the Lord. The dedication is all about the young man.

We came down the aisle arm in arm. I was dressed in a white formal gown, and he had on a white tuxedo and top hat. You do not see this ceremony often, but if anyone ever gets a chance to see this, take it. I only had two rehearsals, and there was no stress involved. I got through this occasion very well with no problems.

During my junior and senior years at the academy, there was no meeting anyone. No prom, and no real graduation. In my senior year, my headaches came more often than usual. I had started to become paranoid about my illness. Every time something happened, I thought I might need surgery again. I knew I had to stop the false alarms. I would go to the hospital. Once inside, I would undergo the entire series of dangerous radiologic tests, and then I would be all right. I was always happy there would be nothing wrong, but when will I know if the alarm is real?

My church was having a debutante ball. I thought this might somehow take the place of the prom that I never had. It did not. I did enjoy dressing up in my beautiful white princess dress that my aunt made for me. I had danced and dined with my date, and I also danced with my dad. That was nice. Everyone was so beautiful, and enjoyed the whole night.

I had another blackout headache exactly three weeks after the debutante ball. One early morning at about 2:00 a.m., I got up to go to the bathroom, turned on the light, and felt a bad headache knock me to the floor. That is the only thing I remember about that morning. My mom was there when I came to. I asked her what happened. She told me that she heard me call out to her, so she came. We went to the hospital just to see if anything was wrong. The doctor informed us that there was no problem with the shunt. This really stressed me out. I started to wonder, when will this happen again? Not only did I pass out for a few seconds, I also had no energy for at least two days. The bad headache that I had in New Orleans was second to the spells I was having at that moment.

When I start to stress out about the blackouts that seem to happen to me more and more, I will sometimes read Bible verses. I like to read Hebrews 11:1-10.

1. Now faith is the substance of things hope for, and the evidence of things not seen.
2. For by it elders obtained a good report

3. Through faith we understand that the worlds were framed by the world of God, so that things which are seen were not made of things which do appear.
4. By faith Abel offered unto God a more sacrifice than Cain, by which the obtained witness that he was righteous, God testifying of his gifts, and by it he being dead yet speaketh.
5. By faith Enoch was translated that he should not see death, and before his translation he had this testimony, that he pleased God.
6. But without faith it is impossible to please Him, for he that cometh to God must believe that He is a Rewarder to those that diligently seek Him.
7. By faith Noah, being warned of God of things not seen as yet, moved with fear, prepared an ark to the savings of his house; by which He condemned the world, and became heir of the righteousness which is by faith.
8. By faith Abraham, when he was called to go out into a place which he should after receive an inheritance, obeyed, and he went out, not knowing whither he went.
9. By faith he sojourned in the land of promise, as in a strange country, dwelling in tabernacles with Isaac and Jacob, the Heirs with him of the same promise.
10. For he looked for a city which hath foundations, whose builder and maker is God.

I finally began to see how different kinds of stress could trigger the headaches. I have yet to be able to control the situations. I did, however, manage to see one coming. My mom's mother died, and I remembered the last stress I had from a death in the family. So, when this grandmother, whom I loved very much, passed away, I look it easy. I did not tire myself out, and I did not sit at the funeral home all day. I just tried to remember the special times. Even with all the precautions I took, I still got another headache, but it only lasted one day.

I had made an appointment to see my doctor, because I was having smaller headaches more often. My mom drove me to that doctor's appointment, as she did all the time. Upon arriving for my appointment, my mom parked in the hospital garage. We walked to the signal light and waited for the light to change. I saw the light change, and then I felt a headache. Then my mom was holding me on the ground. She told me that I was out for about three to five seconds. That headache came on me suddenly and quickly. We had to take about three to five minutes to get things together so that we could continue on for my appointment. When I arrived at the doctor's office, I told the neurologist what had just happened. She examined me, and ran lab tests, and still saw nothing wrong.

This time, I started to trip again. What is going on? Am I sick again, or what? The headaches have gotten worse. They don't seem to give me any kind of warning. It appears to me that as I get older, the headaches knock me on the floor; I black out at least three to four seconds. And when I do come back, it feels as though I was out for a long time. I also noticed that when I watch different movies or read stories, I seem to have difficulty understanding what I have read, what the story was about, or who the main character was. Things like that. My memory loss negatively affected my life. In times like this, I sometimes like to refer to Isaiah.

Isaiah 53:5 - But He was wounded for our Transgression. He was bruised for our iniquities, the chastisement of our Peace was upon Him, and with His Stripes we are healed.

I don't know if I ever had any kind of control in my life or nobody else's. I have let my disability affect my future.

I am taking control now. I have never written anything in the form of an autobiography, a book, or anything else. However this autobiography turns out, I believe someone will be able to relate and understand their own life a little bit better.

I am Kacee, a twenty-eight year old woman. I am the daughter of Joseph and Cathy. I am also a sister, niece, auntie, and author. My ambition is to someday become a motivational speaker.

As of now, I am unsure that I will ever lead a normal life, whatever a normal life is supposed to feel like or be. I don't know if I will ever have a real date or even a real boyfriend. I pray that the Lord will provide. It has been very difficult for me to try to figure out what I should be doing with my life. I have been writing this autobiography since 2002. I wrote just so much, and then I stopped, because I was not sure if I should continue to write again.

I felt as though my autobiography was going nowhere, because my life, I felt, was going nowhere.

I searched the computer to see if there was someone with the same type of disability who was close to my age, or even who had life experiences similar to mine. I felt as though I should have some kind of connection to these people with the same disability, people that I have never met. I also felt as though these people would somehow be able to validate me as a real person in some way. I don't feel that way anymore.

I was never able to locate anyone online either. I was lonely for communication. I wanted to relate to someone like me. However, since I am unable to relate to anyone, maybe somehow, someone may in some way be able to relate to me, someday.

I want to rise above this disability, and continue on to what I will be happy doing in life. This is why I decided to finish my story.

I am no longer dwelling in the past. I am living for the future.

THE END

www.ingramcontent.com/pod-product-compliance
Lightning Source LLC
Chambersburg PA
CBHW072014280526
45788CB00005B/2047

* 9 7 8 1 5 4 5 1 2 5 0 9 0 *